Detox: 3 Simple Steps to Regain Your Health

The Simplest Path to Feeling Energized and Alive Without Going to the Gym or Changing Your Diet

By Dr. Richard A. Reiner, DC PA

1st Edition 2014
Copyright © 2014 by Dr. Richard A. Reiner, DC PA

ISBN-13: 978-06923096-9-8
ISBN-10: 0692309691

Published by:
Reiner Chiropractic & Wellness Center
www.ReinerChiro.com

Edited by:
Jennifer-Crystal Johnson
www.JenniferCrystalJohnson.com

Disclaimer: The Publisher and the Author make no representations or warranties with respect to the accuracy or completeness of the contents of this work and specifically disclaim all warranties, including without limitation warranties of fitness for a particular purpose. No warranty may be created or extended by sales or promotional materials. The advice and strategies contained herein may not be suitable for every situation. This work is sold with the understanding that the Publisher is not engaged in rendering legal, accounting, medical, or other professional services. If professional or medical assistance is required, the services of a competent professional person, such as the Author, should be sought.

Neither the publisher nor the Author shall be liable for damages arising here. Just because an organization or website is referred to in this work as a citation and/or a potential source of further information does not mean that the Author or the Publisher endorses the information the organizations or websites may provide or recommendations it may make. Further, readers should be aware that Internet websites listed in this work may have changed or disappeared between the time this work was written and when it is read.

Printed in the United States of America.

*This book is dedicated to every person
who has ever felt fatigued, tired, and thought there
must be a way to feel better again.*

About Dr. Richard A. Reiner & His Ultimate Body Cleanse and Detoxification Program

Dr. Reiner has a strong passion for helping people feel better and healthier.

Dr. Reiner researched and reached out to experts from all over the country for over two years to develop his unique Body Cleanse and Detoxification Program.

Up until creating the program, Dr. Reiner specialized in traumatic and sports injuries. He was the team chiropractor for the Florida Bobcats of the NFL Arena Football League for three years, team chiropractor for the West Palm Beach CBA team, and personal chiropractor to heavyweight boxer David Tua, as well as working with many other professional athletes in South Florida. For years, Dr. Reiner's main focus was helping athletes.

In 2000, a very close cousin of Dr. Reiner living in New Orleans developed stomach and esophageal cancer. While his cousin was undergoing chemotherapy and other treatments, he asked Dr. Reiner, "Is there anything that you could do to help me?" Dr. Reiner replied, "I'm a musculoskeletal specialist. I don't deal with internal problems." Unfortunately, his cousin passed away.

Not long after his cousin died, Dr. Reiner's daughter's childhood best friend's mother developed breast cancer, and as she was going through her treatments, she *also* asked him, "Is there anything you could do to help me?" Again he replied, "I'm a musculoskeletal guy."

Dr. Reiner felt like somebody was sending him a message to also help people with their internal health instead of just their musculoskeletal problems.

So he decided to start researching about the internal problems of the body and noninvasive procedures to help the body heal naturally. The first thing he learned about was far infrared saunas and their benefits. He learned about lymphatic drainage massages and about the detox footbath, which led him to incorporating the use of enhanced air (oxygen) to further help people. There's a chiropractic neurologist who specializes in dealing with post-stroke patients, and he had been helping them with enhanced air therapy.

Dr. Reiner continued reading about different specializations for healing the body. Additionally, he reached out to many other doctors. There's one doctor who is an infectious disease specialist in the Seattle area, and he talked to her many times about different things that she was doing to help her patients.

There was also a naturopathic specialist who introduced him to certain treatments. He was in Tallahassee, Florida, and another one was in Dallas. Dr. Reiner started meeting and talking to different specialists all over the United States who would say, "Let me give you the name of somebody else who might be able to give you more information."

As Dr. Reiner's knowledge increased, he spent two years trying different things, putting this treatment protocol together, and working with patients until he was finally able to come up with a very concrete program.

Because of the people he knew who passed away because of cancer, he had a strong incentive and passion to perfect a program to help people with their health.

Dr. Reiner's Ultimate Body Cleanse and Detoxification Program treats the body naturally and gives it direction; that's really the key.

Rather than masking the symptoms and telling you to try different products that may or may not work, Dr. Reiner always says, "I don't know what products could work for anybody; I can't tell you the specifics of any particular product, but I can tell you that if you remove the barrier preventing the body from absorbing proper nutrients, then the body has a chance of getting back to health."

That's why Dr. Reiner talks about removing those barriers to poor health. Once the barriers are removed, if you want to take a certain product and you think it will make you feel better, that product at least has an opportunity to work. If the cells and pores in your body are clogged due to toxic build up over time, it doesn't matter what you take; you're not going to properly absorb the nutrients.

Remove the barrier and you can start to heal. Dr. Reiner can consult with you about which treatments may be more or less effective for you.

Dr. Reiner was featured in HERLIFE Magazine in the South Florida October 2014 edition:

http://www.herlifemagazine.com/southflorida/

The article can be viewed here:

http://go.epublish4me.com/ebook/ebook?id=10079924#/34

Dr. Reiner's Background

Dr. Reiner earned his Bachelor's Degree at Ohio State University and did his graduate work at Life Chiropractic College in Marietta, Georgia. He served in the US Army and the US Army National Guard. He is board certified by the National Board of Chiropractic Examiners and has been in private practice since 1982 in West Palm Beach, Florida.

When Dr. Reiner was in undergraduate school, he majored in Systems Analysis research. After he graduated college, he went into the Army and had a minor training incident where his back was slightly injured. Rather than take medication, somebody recommended that he see a chiropractor.

He went twice, got two adjustments, and felt great afterward. When he got out of the service, Dr. Reiner decided to become a product of the product so to speak, because he was very impressed with chiropractic, the philosophy, and how it helps people. He moved to Marietta, Georgia and enrolled at Life Chiropractic College. When he graduated, he moved to West Palm Beach, Florida, where he is currently practicing. Becoming a chiropractor was the best career move Dr. Reiner ever made.

Professional Organizations:

- American Chiropractic Association (ACA).
- ACA Councils on Orthopedics and Sports Medicine.
- Florida Chiropractic Association.
- Palm Beach County Chiropractic Society, Vice President: 1987-1988, 1989-1990, 1990-1991, 1991-1992.
- Insurance Relations Committee Chairman: 1988-1989.
- Parker Chiropractic Research Foundation.
- Foundation of Chiropractic Education and Research.

Other Organizations:

- Humana Gold Plus Plan: PPO Provider.
- Blue Cross/Blue Shield of Florida: PPO Provider.
- Florida Bobcats Arena NFL: Team Chiropractor, 1996-1999.
- WBA/WBC: Personal Chiropractor for David Tua, Heavyweight Boxer.
- Hippocrates Health Institute: Instructor.

Civic Activities:

- Kiwanis Club – Charter Member, Wellington.
- Exchange Club – Charter Member, Wellington.

Postgraduate Education:

- X-Ray Interpretation of Spinal and Skeletal Disorders, Dr. Russell Ehard; 100 hours.
- International College of Applied Kinesiology, Dr. Kenneth Feder; 100 hours.
- International College of Applied Kinesiology, Advanced Studies, Dr. George Goodheart; 60 hours.
- Use of AMA's Guides to the Evaluation of Permanent Impairment, Dr. Stanley Kaplan; 100 hours.
- Treatment of Low Back Disorders, Dr. James Cox; 60 hours.
- Tortipelvis and Scoliosis, Dr. Fred Barge; 40 hours.
- Manipulation Under Anesthesia, Texas Chiropractic College; 40 hours.
- Sports Injuries, Dr. Leroy Perry; 24 hours.
- UFHEC, School of Medicine, Santo Domingo, D.R.; 3 years.
- Physician Certification Program for Worker's Compensation

To schedule a free consultation with Dr. Reiner, call 561-689-4700 or visit www.ReinerChiro.com. Be sure to mention this book to receive your complimentary consultation.

A Message from Dr. Reiner

In the 30 years of operating my private practice, I noticed there were more and more patients who felt sick, tired, or fatigued. As a result of wanting to help my patients feel better, I was on a mission to develop a unique system to help them achieve better health.

While I cannot claim this system will cure illnesses such as cancer, fibromyalgia, Epstein Barr, arthritic conditions, insomnia, chronic fatigue syndrome, chronic neck and back pain, etc., I *can* tell you the techniques we use in this body cleanse system have helped some of our patients *with* these illnesses feel better. As I tell all my patients, this unique body cleanse system may or may not work for you, but it is worth trying.

For example, I helped a gentleman using a cane to ambulate due to MS. After two sessions, the patient was able to stop using his cane for months… *just from two sessions.* Again, I do not claim to cure MS as it's a neurological problem, but the patient had such relief from my Body Cleanse and Detoxification Program; it was amazing.

I had another gentleman who was referred to me from Philadelphia. This patient was so impressed with my program that he purchased a condo in our area so he could come whenever he wanted.

I had a woman who called from Seattle and asked me about anyone in the Seattle area offering my program and I told her, "No, I don't know anybody in Seattle who does anything like this." So she called me back and asked, "Are you anywhere near Royal Palm Beach? I have a cousin who lives there." Royal Palm Beach is about five miles away. She called her cousin and spent a week with her. She came, had three sessions, and felt great.

The mother of a medical supply specialist I know lives in Clearwater, which is on the west coast of Florida. She's been suffering from health issues that nobody could define. She went to the Mayo Clinic. Her insurance paid thousands of dollars for her evaluations and treatments and they told her, "We don't know what's wrong. Maybe it's psychosomatic. When you go home, get checked out." Obviously, that's not what she wanted to hear. She told her son and he said, "Come spend next week with me at my house," which was not far from my office. She came for three sessions on Monday, Wednesday, and Friday, and went back to work the following week. She called me and said, "I don't understand everything you did even though you explained it to me, but this is the best I've felt in years; I'm so happy I came."

Another woman from the Fort Lauderdale area, which is about an hour drive from our office, was diagnosed with fibromyalgia. She was a chemistry researcher with a Ph.D. working in the pharmaceutical industry. Due to being around drugs and chemicals for so many years, apparently they got absorbed into her body and she developed fibromyalgia to the point where she could hardly function – her muscle and joint pain was traumatic, and she was only in her late 30's, a young mother with two young boys. Her rheumatologist told her, "Listen, there's nothing I can do for you other than prescribe steroids." That was the typical treatment, either prednisone and/or cortisone. He also recommended that she apply for social security disability. She said, "I don't want to do that. I really want to go back to work." He said, "I don't see how you can."

Well, her mother knew somebody affiliated with our office, so she referred her here. She drove up from Fort Lauderdale after I spoke to her and I said, "Try one session and see how you feel." She had one session. She gave me a hug afterwards and said, "Right now I have no pain at all. This was incredible, can I come back?" And I said, "Of course."

So, she drove twice a week for care for about a month. Now she comes in three times a year, just to maintain what she's done, and already she's in the job market looking to get back to work; she has no desire to even think about disability.

Again, I don't claim to cure cancer or anything else, but I'm helping people return to proper health. Most people who suffer from conditions such as fibromyalgia watch television ads, and one of the ads that promote a fibromyalgia "treatment" is Lyrica. When you see a Lyrica commercial, one of the so-called "side effects" is a suicidal tendency. Sure, Lyrica will help you, but do you want to risk being suicidal? Of course not!

Many of the commercials today, when they talk about the benefits of these so-called treatments, they have a bigger list of side effects than benefits. They shouldn't be called side effects. A side effect would be if you stub your toe and it turns black and blue because you stubbed it. What they're talking about are different types of negative effects.

An effect would be a response to taking a certain medication. They'll say, "Well, this could happen to you." Those described in commercials are negative effects of the medication. When they say side effect, they are trying to minimize it. "Oh, it's only a side effect, it's no big deal." No, it's a *negative* effect; it really is a big deal. People die from these so-called "side effects."

Another patient I helped was a young man in his 40's who was an athlete when he was in high school. He was captain of his high school football team until he was in the bottom of a pile up in his senior year and had multiple fractures in his right ankle. That ended his high school football career, and he had been hoping to get a scholarship to play football in college. He was a good athlete, and that ended abruptly.

He did go to college and got his degree. He works near my office and I saw him limping one day. He said, "Once in a while my right ankle really has a lot of pain. There's inflammation there because of this old injury."

We started doing the ionic detox foot bath with him and it pulled the inflammation out. While he could only do light workouts at the gym before, now he's running on the treadmill. He said he hardly ever has any ankle pain anymore and that these treatments have been life-changing for him to get back into shape.

Recently, I had a couple of patients who were involved in auto accidents where the airbag deployed, and if you've ever seen anybody who had an airbag deploy, you'll oftentimes see burn marks on their forehead or their forearms where they were hit because of the force.

These patients were concerned because of the bruising the air bag left, so I said, "Listen, we're going to go in the far infrared sauna." Because far infrared rays have healing properties, I put them in there for half an hour. They come back the next day and there's barely a blemish on them. It just gets rid of that potential scar tissue that could be there and replaces it with healthy tissue.

It's just amazing to see the difference, and I know that if it helps to heal externally within 24 hours, it also helps the body heal those injured tissues internally. We have a whole arsenal of different types of treatments that you will not typically find in other offices.

I had another gentleman who was 70 years old and had a right knee problem. His meniscus was partially torn, but he loved to golf. He hadn't been able to golf in six months since having a surgical procedure because he still had knee pain. A friend referred him to me to do the detox footbath. We pulled inflammation out of his knee, I did electrotherapy on it, I adjusted it, and he walked out of the office pain free.

He called me a week later and said, "Hey, I just played two rounds of golf and my knee didn't bother me. I was told I may need to have another surgical procedure on my knee, but forget that." He drove over from Naples, Florida, which is a good two hour drive. He came over just to do this procedure. He wouldn't have driven two hours unless he thought there was an alternative to doing another surgical procedure, and we exceeded his initial expectation.

There's a family of five brothers and sisters that live in Tampa. Again, that's on the other side of the state. They come twice a year as a family to do detox sessions with us. They stay overnight at their aunt's house in West Palm Beach, then drive home the next day. They've been doing this for a couple of years now and they love it.

I had another female patient who works in the dental department at the VA Hospital. She first came to me in October because she was recovering from breast cancer. She was having a lot of upper extremity pain where they did chemotherapy and radiation procedures on her. When she first came to us, she needed a cane to walk because of the weakness in her body. She told me the last time she was home, which is Chicago, it was over Labor Day – she was in a wheelchair because she couldn't walk. Then, her family saw her again over Christmas.

I started treating in October, November, and part of December, about two and a half months of care. When her family saw her, they expected her to come with a wheel chair or a cane, and she came walking off the plane, waving to everybody and ready to go dancing; they were in total shock. They looked at her and said, "My God, look at you. What have you done these past couple of months? How did you do it?" She said, "I got a new doctor that's treating me with this body cleanse." They just looked at the results and were flabbergasted.

These are typical results of patients who go through my Body Cleanse and Detoxification Program.

Helping patients and changing lives is really what keeps me motivated and excited. When people come to me with different health issues and say, "I don't know if you can help me. I've been to so many doctors, and some can help me while some never really did much." I tell them right up front, "I don't know if I can help you, either. All I can say is try a session and tell me how you feel." And when they finish, they ask, "When can I come back?" That's the most common question I hear.

This program I developed is what has given me renewed energy and vigor for practicing in my profession because I am now offering something that nobody else does and we're achieving such positive results and helping so many people.

I went to school to become a doctor. I developed a passion to help people achieve better health. I have the opportunity to help many people, and that is why I'm practicing.

There is no challenge that I'm not up for. I am willing to help anybody who feels that they've gone the medical route, they're sick and tired of feeling like nobody can help them, and now suddenly we're giving them a new lease on life.

Without a doubt, helping people feel better is my favorite part of being a chiropractor. When you see a smile on somebody's face after they have been suffering and they say thank you. Or when you get a hug from somebody that says, "Oh my God, I was told I may need surgery; now I don't." That's the real satisfaction.

I wrote this book to share some success stories from patients and give you an overview of our exclusive Body Cleanse and Detoxification Program as well as our practice.

My staff absolutely loves doing the Body Cleanse and Detox Program. They get excited when they see the results people have, and the more people come in to do it, the happier they are. To them, that's what makes working with me worthwhile.

When you're stressed, your body goes through physiological change because there are three forms of stress: mental, physical, and chemical or emotional. It could be a combination or just one that causes the body to feel uncomfortable. For example, physical stress – you fall down, you hurt yourself, or you're in a car accident. Your body is sore and in pain, you experienced a traumatic event. Mental stress could be your job, your family, anything on your mind that could affect your body and your physiology. Chemical or emotional stress could be eating food that doesn't agree with you, smoking, drinking excessive alcohol, or taking drugs; these could all have a chemical effect on the body. Any one of them, or a combination, can cause the body to start to wear down. What we're doing with my program is trying to remove that wear and tear obstacle and rebuild, and help your body get back to where it needs to be. Everybody should try my program because we all have stress in our lives.

I urge you to schedule a free consultation to see me at our West Palm Beach location by calling 561-689-4700. Make sure to mention this book to receive your complimentary consultation.

I look forward to meeting you!

To your good health,

Dr. Reiner

Success Stories from Actual Patients

Below you'll find some success stories submitted by some of Dr. Reiner's actual patients.

★★★★★

I was referred to Dr. Reiner by "A Season to Share." I repeatedly suffered from ovarian cancer that kept coming back. I needed monthly blood work to check my levels. Dr. Reiner treated me for one month before I went back to the lab for blood work; they called me to repeat the test, which showed my body was cancer free. This was truly a holiday blessing.

-Yvette A.

★★★★★

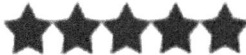

My mother had been diagnosed with cancer and receiving chemotherapy treatments, causing her extreme discomfort in her legs, lethargy, and a loss of appetite. She visited a friend who is a patient of Dr. Reiner, who suggested that she visit his office about his wellness program to address her symptoms. When she returned to NJ, I could not believe the transformation. She was much more like her old self. Dr. Reiner and his staff went above and beyond to provide my mother with the best care.

-Scott M.

-

★★★★★

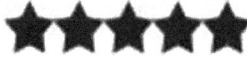

I was a research chemist when I developed severe fibromyalgia through exposure to many chemicals. My family doctor suggested that I apply for disability benefits, but I wasn't ready to stop working. Dr. Reiner's treatments helped me overcome my pain and I'm enjoying life again.

-Natalie T.

★★★★★

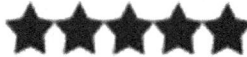

I am a new client, but to tell you the truth, I wish I had found Dr. Reiner and his staff years ago. When I leave the office I feel WONDERFUL and look forward to the next appointment. With swelling in my feet and legs, the foot detox has helped me so much. The massage and sauna is a PLUS for getting all those nasty toxins out of by body. I would HIGHLY recommend giving Dr. Reiner's office a chance. You won't be disappointed, I promise!!!

-Alma R.

★★★★★

I was referred to Dr. Reiner by two of my co-workers about eight months ago. I've had chronic neck issues and insomnia for many years. Since I have been doing the detox, my pain level has decreased and I can sleep better at night. I am so grateful to Dr. Reiner and his staff. They always make me feel comfortable and I always leave the office feeling very relaxed.

-Marina S.

★★★★★

I was referred to Dr. Reiner for treatment of back pain and overall tiredness. Once I started care, I realized that I was receiving much more than regular chiropractic adjustments. His total wellness program included a wonderful body cleanse and detox that not only helped me overcome back pain but it made me feel so much better. I now have energy that keeps me going all the time. I now have my daughter going and she loves it, too. Thank you, Dr. Reiner.

-Maria L.

★★★★★

Dr. Reiner has been a wonderful help to me since 2009. He specializes in being caring and professional. I had problems with my lower back and my shoulders. Dr. Reiner listened to me describe my discomfort and then went to work on making me feel better. He gave practical tips that really helped. I would highly recommend Dr. Reiner for all chiropractic needs. Thanks!

-Cathy P.

★★★★★

I was in search of a chiropractic/holistic doctor due to heavy metal poisoning. Getting in touch with Dr. Reiner has been my biggest lifesaver; I've gone for one treatment already and feel a HUGE difference! Looking forward to my upcoming detox sessions! He truly cares about your wellbeing and health!

-Melissa H.

★★★★★

I worked as a post-operative nurse for over 10 years and was always tired after a 12 hour shift. At least once a month I got sick due to exhaustion and exposure to sick patients. After starting Dr. Reiner's Body Cleanse Program, my resistance level picked up; I hardly ever get sick and do not miss days from work.

-Anni H.

★★★★★

I was diagnosed with mold poisoning after exposure at work. My doctor sent my lab tests to the CDC in Atlanta and they reported a near fatal reading. I was placed on Dr. Reiner's "Intensive Care" treatment for one month. Lab work was repeated and sent to the CDC and it came back; barely a trace of mold remained in my system. Dr. Reiner's detox program is amazing.

-Michelle M.

★★★★★

I work out regularly at the gym. Occasionally, my body stresses out and I feel lethargic and become susceptible to getting a cold or flu-like symptoms. Whenever I feel this way, I go to Dr. Reiner for the far infrared sauna and detox footbath, and within a short time, I feel great.

-Michael A.

★★★★★

I suffered with fibromyalgia for years. It interfered with my ability to work and made me miserable whenever I traveled. I was referred to Dr. Reiner for a series of treatments. I was amazed at how well I felt after just the first treatment. I highly recommend Dr. Reiner's Body Cleanse/Detox program.

-Sunny Q.

★★★★★

I selected his office because of location and am so glad I did. He takes his time, explains everything, and his method has made my recovery so much faster than I ever expected. I highly recommend him!!!

-Ronald R.

★★★★★

I really love the entire detox package. After my therapy, I felt different. My skin felt really smooth and I loved the overall feeling.

-Marisha H.

★★★★★

As a snowbird coming from NY, I received a brochure on the body cleansing and detox program at Dr. Reiner's practice. After this treatment I felt more rejuvenated at my age of 71. Gratitude to Dr. Reiner.

-Steven V.

★★★★★

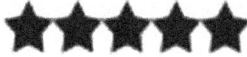

One year ago I was diagnosed with stage four breast cancer with metastasis to bone. My hips and shoulder were affected; I needed assistance with a cane for six months before and after my radiation. Lactic acid build-up in both legs and hips caused excruciating pain in the day and worse at night. Dr. Reiner put me on an intensive care treatment. After just two weeks, I got rid of the pain and the lactic acid in my legs dissipated.

-Dion J.

The purpose of these actual patients' success stories is to show you how Dr. Reiner's Body Cleanse and Detoxification Program has helped them. There are no guarantees that the system will help you, but it is certainly worth a complimentary consultation with Dr. Reiner to learn more.

To schedule your complimentary consultation with Dr. Reiner, call 561-689-4700 and mention this book.

What is Dr. Reiner's Non-Invasive Body Cleanse & Detox Program… and Why Does it Work?

We live in a world today where toxins exist in abundance. They surround us in the air we breathe, the food we eat, and through stress. Therefore, we have a need to regularly detoxify on a mental, physical, and emotional level in order to regain and maintain the balance in our life. Most of us only realize we are toxic when we don't feel good, and even then we aren't always able to identify what's wrong. Dr. Reiner has created what he believes is the ultimate in body cleansing and detox programs.

You shower and brush your teeth on a regular basis; why not clean yourself from the inside? You are internally susceptible to the same toxins that affect you on the outside, and now you have an opportunity to clean your body from within.

Have you ever taken a bite out of an apple and set it down? What happens to the apple after a while? Obviously, the apple turns brown. That's called oxidation, and what causes the oxidation is free radicals in the air.

Well, guess what? We're breathing those same free radicals. So if you see what it's doing to the apple, you know it's doing something to your body as well, and it's not necessarily good. We also drink and eat food processed with preservatives and other chemicals (GMOs) which contribute to the buildup of toxins in our body.

Another name for free radicals is oxidants.

Today, the buzzword is *antioxidants*. Everybody wants to eat blueberries and strawberries and drink smoothies to get these antioxidants. But think about it logically. How many antioxidant products do you think you would have to consume to counter breathing 24/7? Can you eat and drink as much as you breathe? It's impossible.

If you tried to eat and drink as much as you breathe, you'd be big enough to have your own zip code. It just doesn't work. When you're not feeling good or you feel lethargic, there's an accumulation of toxins that have built up in your body. Perhaps you'll go to your family doctor and they'll prescribe medication for you, hoping it will make you feel better, or you may want to go the so-called "natural route" and go to a health food store and buy some kind of colon cleansing product to make you feel good and clean things out.

But over time, your body does accumulate these oxidants or toxins, and they begin to affect the cells and the pores in the organs of your body. And over time, they accumulate and clog these cells and pores and organs, so whatever you take is not necessarily going to be absorbed; it just passes through your system.

The organ responsible for filtering toxins is the liver. When was the last time you cleaned your filter? Can you imagine if you never cleaned the air conditioning filter in your house or the oil filter in your car? Do you think they would work properly? If you choose not to clean your liver or just ignore it, toxins will accumulate in it, eventually saturating the organ and causing it to overflow toxins into surrounding tissues and organs, preventing proper circulation. Stagnation occurs, leading to cellular death. With cellular death, the body's pH changes and becomes acidic.

Toxins can only survive and proliferate in an acidic environment. The way to regain healthy tissues is by eliminating the acidity and changing the body's pH to an alkaline one. How do we do this?

If you have a clogged sink, are you going to throw more stuff in the sink expecting that the extra weight will push through the pipes and then it miraculously starts to drain? Of course not. You have to "Roto-Rooter" the sink to let it drain. That's what Dr. Reiner has accomplished with his Ultimate Body Cleanse & Detoxification Program: a natural "Roto-Rooter" for the body.

With Dr. Reiner's program, you are getting to the core of common health issues because he is also doing pH balancing, which is very important. We do a pH litmus on everybody before they start. 98% of the people who start are acidic. Diseases can only survive when the body is in an acidic pH environment. You change the body's environment, make it alkaline, and most disease processes cannot survive in an alkaline body.

That's what makes Dr. Reiner's program unique, and this is why and how it works.

We start with a Lymphatic Drainage Massage to increase lymphatic flow in the body, moving stagnant fluids to reduce swelling and inflammation. Next we use the Far Infrared Sauna that emits waves into your body to stimulate cellular metabolism and break up water molecules which hold toxins, allowing the body to expel those toxins through perspiration. Finally, we do the Ionic Detox Foot Bath. The water goes through electrolysis to become negatively ionized. These negative ions are absorbed by the body, neutralize the positive ones (free radicals), and release them.

We combine this with enhanced air, which heightens the release of toxins. After all, we breathe polluted air, causing oxygen deprivation. By adding enhanced air, your body becomes energized and it helps push toxins out faster.

The ionic footbath is by far the most visual part of the treatment. Your feet are placed in a shallow pan of warm water with a module that releases negative ions. The treatment lasts 30 minutes. We start with clear tap water, and by the end of the session, the water turns brown, just like the oxidized apple, and toxins have been removed from your body. Your body is now energized and stronger. You feel relaxed, lighter, and experience a greater sense of well-being.

Step 1 – Lymphatic Drainage Massage

We start off with a lymphatic drainage massage. The reason we do this type of massage is because most of the debris your body accumulates travels throughout your lymphatic system. If it gets clogged or blocked, it's not circulating, so our massage therapist, who is certified specifically in lymphatic massage, begins to get the lymph system flowing. After half an hour, when circulation is restored, you want to start to remove the toxins.

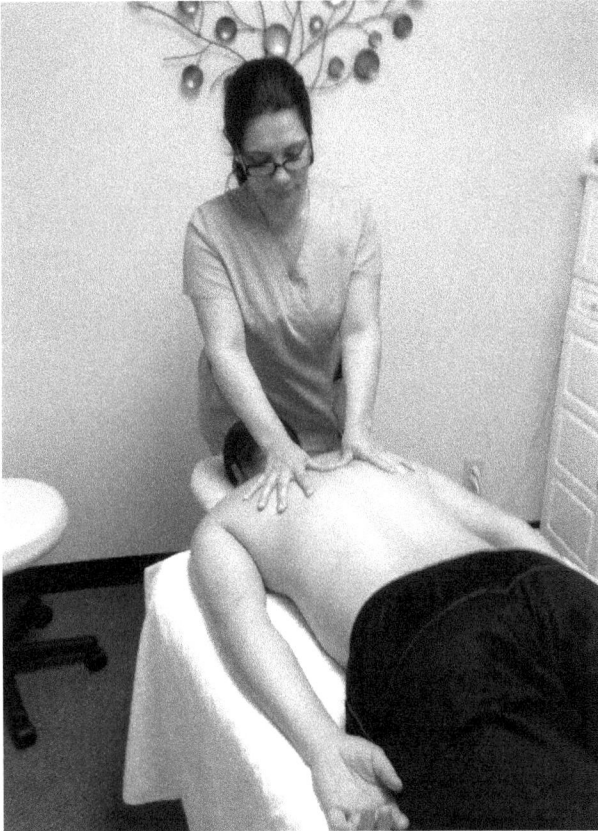

Step 2 – Far Infrared Sauna

Next you go into the far infrared sauna. A far infrared sauna is very different from a regular sauna. A regular sauna that you might see in a gym is like a hot box. It's about 180 degrees, you go in there and you perspire, but 98% of what you perspire is just water coming out from your cells.

A regular sauna works on the same principles as an oven. You have to preheat the oven in order to cook your food, and it heats from the outside in.

The far infrared sauna works in principle more like a microwave oven, as it works from the inside out.

First of all, the far infrared rays mimic the healthy rays of the sun. Unlike the ultraviolet rays that can cause cancer, the far infrared rays are healthy. They penetrate approximately two inches sub-dermal – underneath the surface of the skin – and that's where water molecules bind with toxins. This creates cellular metabolism and breaks up the water molecules, thus allowing the body to void toxins through perspiration.

These far infrared rays are also good for helping cardiovascular cells, restoring internal organs, and repairing scar tissue. It also benefits your skin and helps promote healing of conditions like eczema and psoriasis, and also helps your hair follicles. The far infrared sauna is good for your muscles, your organs, and your joints. Additionally, we have found that women especially love the fact that it speeds up their metabolism.

After half an hour in the far infrared sauna, your body's going to burn up to 600 calories just passively sitting there; I'm sure you'll agree that it takes a lot of exercise to burn 600 calories.

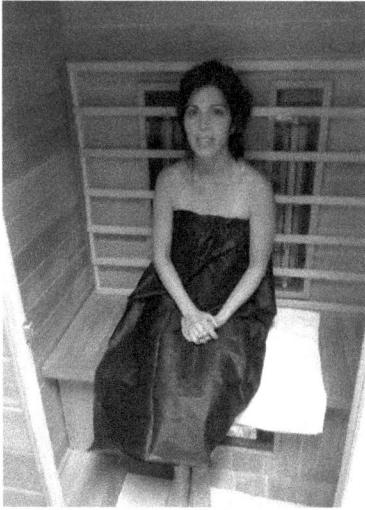

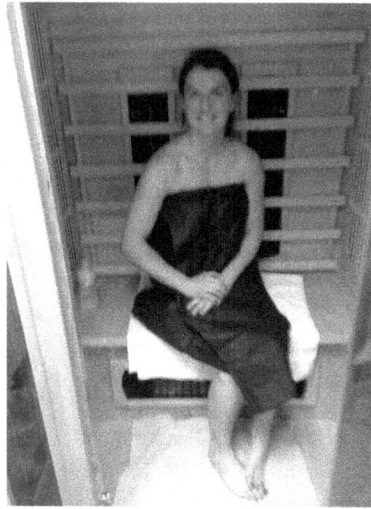

While in the far infrared sauna, you're just sitting there listening to music or reading a magazine and those calories are just falling out of your body.

At this point we've helped you remove external toxins and now we want to remove internal toxins, which we will do in Step 3.

Step 3 – Detox Foot Bath

To remove internal toxins, we do the ionic detox foot bath, where your feet are placed in a shallow pan of warm water with a module that produces negative ions. Negative attracts positive, and the positive ions are the ones that aren't good for you. The negative ions are the healthy ones; the ones that make you feel good. Negative ions are in abundance after it rains and the air has that sweet smell or if you are at the beach when the waves come in and the air has a fresh smell.

Positive ions are associated with stagnation and lack of circulation when the air is heavy and just sits there. The detox foot bath pulls free radicals or oxidants out of your body through your feet. It cleans, balances, and enhances the bio-energy within the body.

Internal cleansing helps liver detoxification, resulting in less body fluid retention, reduced inflammation, a balanced pH, a stronger immune system, and significant pain relief including headaches and arthritis.

The reason your feet are used is because you have about 2000 sweat glands in the bottom of your feet. This concentration of sweat glands is more than in any other part of the body, so it makes for a very easy ionic exchange, and what starts off as clear tap water looks like a bucket of gravy after about half an hour.

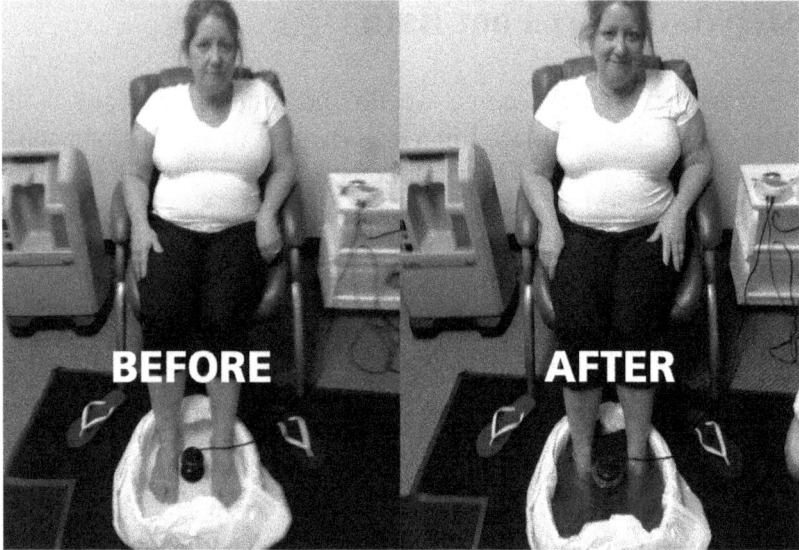

BEFORE **AFTER**

Just like the apple turns brown after half an hour due to oxidation, we're pulling that same oxidation out of your body and into the water. That's why the water turns brown or black, and there are different colors representing different parts of the body.

When the detox foot bath is completed, you stand up and your body has a sense of lightness.

The most common question Dr. Reiner is asked when somebody's doing the foot bath for the first time is, "What did you add to the water to make it dark?" That is by far the most common question. I say, "Nothing. When we started, you saw the water come right out of the faucet. It's clear, isn't it?" Only the module is added to the water with their feet.

When they see it start to work, they ask, "Alright, are you sure there's nothing in this water?" And I say, "Look at the module in the water. What is it connected to? It's a wire. It's not a tube. There's nothing coming through it. Just wires that are plugged into the brains of the outfit, and it's the brains of the outfit that cause the module to produce negative ions. There's no tube, there's nothing added to it. It's all electrical."

The first couple of times people do it, they look down and are mesmerized by what they see. And I'll ask them, "Do you feel anything coming out of your body?" And they say, "No, I just see it." They're just in shock.

The change is coming from the body itself, because when somebody's finished and they stand up, they'll say, "My legs feel lighter, I can walk again, and it feels like I have no pressure...." You know it works.

Now, to add to it, we're giving you enhanced air through the use of an oxygen concentrator. Normally, as we breathe, we're only getting about 21% oxygen. Now, we're giving you 92% enhanced air, and by breathing a higher concentration, it gets into the lower lobes of your lungs that normally don't get the air circulated to it unless you're physically active all the time.

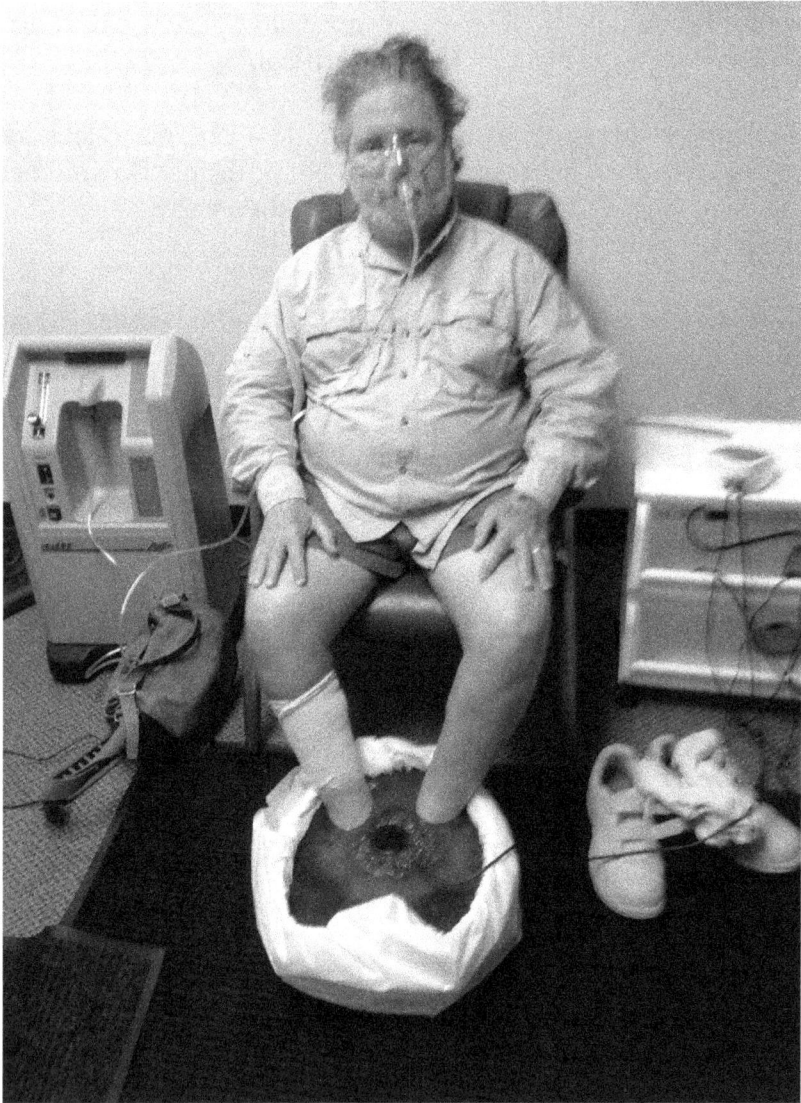

Since most people tend to be more sedentary, they're not really getting that kind of circulation into the lungs

Now we're pushing out this old, stagnant air and replacing it with new, fresh air. As a result, after using the oxygen concentrator, you breathe better. We've helped people with COPD to increase their oxygen intake and feel better.

Nobody does what we do because we developed this format; it works. It's not because Dr. Reiner says it works, it's because the results that he's had with his patients speak for themselves.

Dr. Reiner can't tell you he cures anything, but he will tell you that he has approximately a 90% and higher success rate helping people with conditions such as fibromyalgia, chronic fatigue, Epstein Barr, and many other related situations dealing with arthritic changes.

As we said, you have nothing to lose except bad health. You have everything to gain and feel better. This Body Cleanse and Detox Program is so easy and extremely effective.

Just imagine the benefits when you are *free* from agonizing pain and discomfort, you feel renewed and revitalized… full of energy, ready to take on the day, and your improved health makes you happy.

Feeling healthy is so important. Health is not expensive; it's sickness that affects people physically, emotionally, and financially. We focus on providing patients with a greater quality of life through better health.

To schedule your complimentary consultation in his West Palm Beach office, call 561-689-4700 and mention this book.

How Long Should it Take Before I Feel Better & How Often Should I Do the Program?

The amount of time it takes to feel better really depends on your unique health situation. We have had some patients feel better after one visit; for others it can take several treatments.

If you came to see Dr. Reiner and said, "I work out, I have good muscle tone, and I feel good," and you want to come in occasionally for Dr. Reiner's Body Cleanse and Detoxification Program, that would be fine. We have people come in once every couple months just to feel a little better as Dr. Reiner's Body Cleanse and Detoxification Program helps to take the edge off.

We also have patients come in with real health issues, and they'll come and do Dr. Reiner's Body Cleanse and Detoxification Program twice or three times a week to really help themselves and overcome a lot of their physical ailments.

Again, it depends on your situation. That's why Dr. Reiner does a consultation, because it puts him in a position to know where you are health-wise and what it will take to help you.

Additionally, some patients may not want to do the sauna because they may feel uncomfortable in the heat, so maybe they'll just want to do the massage and the foot bath, or maybe they'll alternate it.

In order to do the entire program, you'd be in the office for almost two hours, and sometimes people don't have two hours to devote to do a whole detox session. Instead, maybe they only have an hour, so they'll just do two of the procedures.

And then, of course, we do the chiropractic adjustment to help loosen up their muscles, joints, and their spine, which complements everything we do.

Today, the largest group of people interested in our Body Cleanse and Detoxification Program are the "Baby Boomers." They have lived an active and healthy life and are not ready to trade in their roller blades for walkers. They want to hold onto their health for as long as possible without worrying about illness or disease that will eventually catch up to them. By far, the most common condition that develops is arthritic changes to the bones and joints of the body. Much of it is due to inflammation in the body and our Body Cleanse and Detoxification Program works best to alleviate the symptoms.

Are There Other Facilities in the West Palm Beach Area That Offer Dr. Reiner's Ultimate Body Cleanse and Detoxification Program?

There may be a couple of facilities that offer just the footbath by itself, but without the enhanced air. There may be a couple of facilities that may offer a far infrared sauna, but without the foot bath or the massage.

Dr. Reiner's office is the only facility he is aware of anywhere that has combined all three of these procedures.

Dr. Reiner spent over two years researching, putting this unique program together, and speaking to experts in different fields within the natural health field all over the country – this was not something he did overnight.

Dr. Reiner spent a long time putting this program together, and when he finally started to do it, he had certain goals in mind, but as he stated before, the results his patients have had far exceeded his wildest expectations.

To schedule your complimentary consultation, call 561-689-4700 and mention this book.

Are There People Who are Restricted From the Program?

There are just a few restrictions as far as who can and cannot do the program. Number one, you should be at least 14 years of age. We do have some parents who bring teenagers in who have attention deficit type problems, and we have been able to help a lot of them.

If a woman is pregnant or nursing, she has to wait until after she finishes her pregnancy or nursing.

If a person has any kind of battery implant, such as a pacemaker, they would not be able to do it.

If a person has had an organ transplant, they would not be able to do it.

These are basically the only restrictions. Just about anybody else can do the Body Cleanse and Detoxification Program.

The only other restriction would be that when they come in, we recommend eating something first. The reason is because for one hour after completing the detox session, you can only drink water because your body is pulling toxins out on a cellular level during the detox, and it will take your body approximately one hour to rehydrate afterward, so while you're rehydrating, you only want to drink water. If you were to eat or drink anything else, that's what you're placing in the cells, which defeats the purpose of the cleanse. After an hour, you're free to go about your normal activities, including diet, without restriction.

Does Insurance Cover the Program?

Once patients come in and find out their insurance covers the treatment, they say, "Where have you been all my life?" That's the kind of response we get.

Some of the federal insurance programs allow multiple treatments per year, so these patients are very excited and become ambassadors of our program. Dr. Reiner has some patients that come in once a week. You know how some people go once a week to massage therapy facility? Well, they'd rather come to Dr. Reiner and receive a full treatment instead of paying a monthly massage fee.

Why is Going to the Chiropractor a Great Alternative to Going to My Medical Doctor?

Most people go to their family doctor when they're not feeling well. They say, "Oh, I've got to make an appointment to see my doctor," and a lot of times the doctor will say, "You know, there really isn't anything I can give you to make you feel better," "Drink more fluids," or, "Cut back on certain foods."

Most people, if they go to the doctor and don't get a prescription feel like, "Hey, why did I bother going? He didn't do his job. I just wasted my copay going to the doctor for nothing." This is how most people think.

Dr. Reiner wants people to have a different attitude when coming to him. He wants people to say, "I'm going there because I want to feel better, and he has a service to provide that's going to make me feel better. I'm going to walk out of Dr. Reiner's office knowing that I'm getting results."

You're going to get results when you come to see Dr. Reiner because he is doing things for you. He is not referring you somewhere else to get another lab test or to see what else could be going on. He knows what's going on, and this is how he is going to help you.

Dr. Reiner offers the public something they're not getting anywhere else.

Can Diet Affect How You Feel?

When a person comes in for their initial consultation and they choose to do the Body Cleanse and Detoxification Program, Dr. Reiner gives them a list of foods that are both alkaline and acidic and, depending upon their pH level, this will determine the diet that is best for them.

If it's very acidic, we encourage them to eat a larger percentage of food from the alkaline chart for the ideal pH level. The pH scale lines run from 0 to 14 and 7 is neutral, right in the middle. The ideal pH for the body is 7.35, which will make it slightly alkaline. However, over 98% of us are more acidic, not because we *want* to be acidic but because most of the foods that we eat cause acidity in the body. Additionally, we are exposed to stress and the air we breathe, all combining to make the body more acidic.

It's a proven fact that when you live near water you are breathing negative ions and it helps your body to balance out more effectively. The further inland you are, where the air is more static, the more positive ions you breathe in and you become more acidic.

The ideal resources for food are natural or organic fruit and vegetables as they are more alkaline. If you have to cook food to eat it, it tends to turn acidic. A popular belief is that citric acid foods such as oranges, grapefruit, lemons, and limes remain acidic, but actually they turn alkaline once they are absorbed into the body. The only fruit that does remain acidic is the cranberry, but we don't eat them often.

As part of your first consultation, Dr. Reiner gives you a list of the most popular alkaline and acidic foods and we encourage you to eat more from the alkaline list to start your pH balancing. He also works with you to help detox the liver because the liver is the filter of the body. You want to clean your filter just like you clean your oil filter in your car or the air conditioning filter in your home. We always have to clean and replace filters. However, you can't replace your liver; it has to work your whole life.

Dr. Reiner doesn't give a full diet plan because not everybody can eat the same food. You may have a food allergy, for instance, and you would not be able to tolerate certain things. So, Dr. Reiner gives you food groupings. He explains that certain oils are easier for your body to digest and which ones to avoid. Additionally, Dr. Reiner talks about trans-fatty acid in nature, which will affect the body in a negative way.

Dr. Reiner talks about GMOs, which is a big buzz word today. They are genetically altered foods that some restaurants use because they find it less expensive than using whole foods.

Whole foods tend to be more expensive and not every store offers them. To purchase these foods you typically have to go to a place like Whole Foods. For instance, fruits that have a hard coating don't really need to be all-natural because pesticides are not going to penetrate through the skin. For example, cantaloupe and watermelon have hard coatings. However, if you are talking about eating lettuce, which doesn't have a coating, you're always better off natural. Overall, try to eat more natural when possible.

In many places, they have green markets on the weekends where many local growers come to sell their products. These products are generally very healthy, natural, and good for you.

Dr. Reiner also encourages you to get fresh fruits, vegetables, or eggs directly from the farm versus the supermarket. Not only can you tell the difference in quality and taste, but overall, farm fresh will be better for you.

Does Dr. Reiner Offer Other Services Besides the Body Cleanse and Detoxification Program?

Just because Dr. Reiner does the Body Cleanse and Detoxification Program doesn't minimize the fact that he is also a chiropractor. Dr. Reiner enjoys providing chiropractic care as well, but he is opening up a whole new venue of health care that you will not find anywhere else.

Dr. Reiner has had a few people come to him and say, "I just want to do the body cleanse. I'm really not interested in getting a chiropractic adjustment." But when they come in and see the other services that he provides, suddenly they're thinking, "Oh, can I get an adjustment, too?"

Dr. Reiner sees a number of people involved in automobile accidents, as these are people who have had traumatic injuries to their body.

Additionally, he sees athletes with sprains, strains, and other injuries. Other patients include people with headaches or maybe they have certain allergies that are affecting their health.

Dr. Reiner sees patients who suffer slip and fall accidents or may be doing gardening and they strain their muscles because they are not used to that type of physical work. From the weekend athletes to the weekend gardeners and anyone who comes to Dr. Reiner for these minor aches and pains, he knows how to treat them quickly for a speedy recovery.

According to the National Institute of Health, approximately 80% of the population will suffer from back pain at some point in their life, but only 10-12% of the population seeks out chiropractic care while the other 80-90% go to their family doctors who generally prescribe muscle relaxants and pain medication and tell people to rest. If you have a pinched nerve, medication cannot un-pinch it. You have to go to a chiropractor who knows how to un-pinch the nerve through adjustments and allow the nerve to become restored to its normal position and then you will feel better.

Dr. Reiner knows how to give you the proper adjustment to give you relief. Sometimes the pain can return unexpectedly. When this occurs, Dr. Reiner will modify the treatment by using therapies first to relax the muscle, and then once you relax the muscle you do the chiropractic adjustment and the body will accept it much more readily and it will help your adjustment hold much longer. At times, depending upon the case and severity of your condition, you may need multiple treatments.

The spine has 24 movable segments. So, if one of these segments is knocked out of place it is going to put pressure on that part of the body. When the nerve has pressure on it, the nerve impulse can only go to one of three places: it goes to a muscle, an organ, or soft tissue. There is nowhere else it can go. So, if that nerve is pinched, it's going to affect the part of the body where it goes. And usually, there's going to be some pain involved. Through adjustments, Dr. Reiner is accelerating the body's ability to improve.

How Often Should Patients Visit Dr. Reiner?

If a patient is being seen for a specific condition such as having been in an automobile accident, they will be placed on a treatment schedule. Some patients come to us on an as-needed basis, which may be once a week, once a month, or once every other month. The number of visits depends upon the condition. Once you feel good, you don't want to be in pain. So, when you come in for a treatment and walk out feeling good, you'll want to come in to keep feeling good.

Other patients see Dr. Reiner only when they need it. For example, you may have bent down and picked up something heavy and felt your back tighten up. Typically, a couple of treatments help resolve the pain and then you are good until the next time.

There isn't one right answer to how often you should see Dr. Reiner as everybody has different needs.

How Do I Meet Dr. Reiner?

To schedule a free consultation with Dr. Reiner, call 561-689-4700 or visit www.ReinerChiro.com. Make sure to mention this book to receive your complimentary consultation.

www.ingramcontent.com/pod-product-compliance
Lightning Source LLC
Chambersburg PA
CBHW050548210326
41520CB00012B/2763